KETOGENIC DIET

The Essential Beginner's Guide to Quick
Weight Loss and Clean Eating

60 Quick and Simple Low Carb Keto Recipes

TYLER SMITH

Table of Contents

Introduction

I want to thank you and congratulate you for getting a copy of, *"Ketogenic Diet: The Essential Beginner's Guide to Quick Weight Loss and Clean Eating"*

This book contains proven steps and strategies on how you can benefit from incorporating the ketogenic diet into your lifestyle. The diet does not only help in your weight loss efforts. More importantly, it will help you achieve good overall health.

To help you get started on the diet, included in the book are easy to follow breakfast, lunch, dinner, and dessert recipes.

Thanks again for getting a copy of this book, I hope you enjoy it!

Chapter 1: Ketogenic Diet Basics

About the Ketogenic Diet

Who says that all types of fat are bad for the health and can be detrimental to your weight loss goals? One of the more popular diets for weight loss today, the ketogenic diet, disproves the misconception.

Truth is, excessive consumption of carbs is the culprit – not fat. So, what exactly is the ketogenic diet?

Also known simply as keto, the ketogenic diet is similar to the low-carb and Atkins diets. It is a diet high in fat and very low in carbs. Basically, the diet involves considerable reduction of carb intake, which is replaced with a high fat intake.

The reduced carb intake will put the body in a metabolic state known as ketosis. When in ketosis, the body becomes a very efficient fat-burning machine. Fat in the liver is also turned into ketones that can supply the brain with energy. Simply put, the body's metabolism is shifted away from carbs in favor of fat and ketones.

Ketogenic diet can help significantly reduce sugar and insulin levels in the blood. Along with increased ketone production, this results to a lot health benefits and improved well-being. These include lowering the risk for serious diseases.

Who can benefit from the Ketogenic Diet?

Ketogenic diet expert Dr. Darag Rennie says that the diet is, in general, safe if done properly. People suffering from the following conditions can benefit from the diet as well:

- Overweight
- Obesity
- Hypertension
- Epilepsy or seizures
- High triglyceride levels
- Metabolic syndrome

However, people afflicted with the following conditions are advised to consult their physician first or take the necessary precautions when considering adopting the ketogenic diet:

- Cancer
- Osteoarthritis
- Dementia
- Polycystic ovary syndrome (PCOS)
- Stroke
- Heart ailments
- Inflamed bowel disease (IBD)
- Irritable bowel syndrome (IBS)

- Autoimmune disorders

- Schizophrenia or bipolar disorder

- Parkinson's disease

- Amyotrophic lateral sclerosis (ALS)

- Attention deficit hyperactivity disorder (ADHD)

- Autism

- Migraine

Ketogenic Diet and Weight Loss

As mentioned, the keto diet is not only effective in promoting better health and well-being. It is also a popular diet to lose weight, and is proven to be more effective than low-fat diets.

The best part is, this diet is so extremely filling that you can forget about counting and strictly tracking your calories. Simply put, keto allows you to lose weight without making you hungry.

If you are on keto diet, you can potentially lose 2 times more excess weight than people on low-fat and calorie-restricted diets. Likewise, you can expect your HDL cholesterol and Triglyceride levels to significantly improve.

There are numerous reasons that make the keto diet superior to low-fat diets for losing weight. For one, keto promotes higher protein consumption that is beneficial in many ways. The diet also causes an increase in ketones, reduced blood sugar levels, and better insulin sensitivity.

Benefits of the Ketogenic Diet

Although weight loss is the inmost popular benefit of the keto diet, it has other health benefits as well.

Weight Loss Benefits

- Increases the body's fat-burning ability – This results in better weight loss. The good news is it happens whether you are at rest or busy with your everyday tasks.

- Burns more calories – Because proteins and fats are converted into energy, more calories are burned.

- Reduces the body's fat storage – This helps eliminate fat build-up and promotes healthy weight loss.

- Less calorie intake – The diet limits your consumption of carbs and other unhealthy food options, effectively limiting your overall calorie intake.

- Improves metabolism – The keto diet helps to curb your appetite, and as a result, weight gain. This is partly due to the increased consumption of protein that facilitates better metabolism.

- Increased insulin sensitivity – Because of your improved metabolism, your body's response to insulin is likewise improved.

Overall Wellbeing

- Diabetes – With its proven ability to lower LDL cholesterol levels, the ketogenic diet is a big help for diabetics. If you maintain low LDL levels consistently for a long time, your risk of contracting poor blood sugar control-related diseases is effectively reduced.

- Heart diseases – The keto diet has the ability to lower your triglyceride levels and prevent arterial build-up that can lead to heart attacks, strokes, and other fatal heart conditions. Keto diet can also improve your body fat and cholesterol levels, and blood pressure, effectively reducing your risk of serious health conditions.

- Cancer – Many studies are being done today on the diet's effect in delaying tumor growth as well as the symptoms that develop as cancer progresses.

- Neurological diseases – The diet can help limit the symptoms caused by various neurological disorders that affect the nervous system and the brain such as Alzheimer's and Parkinson's diseases.

- Metabolic syndrome – The ketogenic diet can considerably decrease insulin resistance. Thus, women with PCOS can expect better weight control and reduced testosterone levels.

- Acne – You may be surprised, but keto diet has a positive effect on skin inflammations and acne. According to studies, less consumption of processed food and sugars promote clearer skin.

For Physical Performance

Although you may feel weak at the start of your journey with the keto diet, you will begin to experience an increase in energy as the days go by. This is because of the transition that your body is going through which has to do with the shift of energy sources – from carbs and sugar to fats.

Various Types of the Ketogenic Diet

The keto diet has different variations. These include:

- Standard Ketogenic Diet or SKD – This type of keto diet is moderate in protein, very low in carb, and high in fat. The ratio is usually 5% carb, 20% protein, and 75% fat.

- Cyclical Ketogenic Diet or CKD – In this type of ketogenic diet, you are allowed more time for higher-carb re-feeds like 5 keto days to be followed by a couple of days with high-carb intake.

- Targeted Ketogenic Diet or TKD – The diet allows adding carbs during your workout days.

- High Protein Ketogenic Diet – Similar to SKD, the diet involves more protein consumption. The more frequently-used ratio is 5% carb, 35% protein, and 60% fat.

While there are several types of ketogenic diets, only the high protein and standard varieties have undergone extensive study and research. Since the targeted and cyclical types of keto diets are comparatively more advanced, these are used mainly by athletes or bodybuilders, and are not commonly recommended for use by regular dieters.

What to Eat and What not to Eat

The keto diet is about healthy food consumption. Here is a list of healthy food you can consume, as well as the type of food you should avoid.

Food to Eat:

Vegetables – The best veggies for the keto diet are the non-starchy types that grow above-ground.

- Cruciferous veggies like kale, radish and kohlrabi

- Leafy greens like Swiss chard, bok choy, lettuce, spinach, chard, chive, radiccio, and endive, among others

- Other veggies such as cucumber, celery stalk, summer squash, and bamboo shoots

Fats – This means the healthy kinds of fat.

- Fats from grass-fed animals or organic sources

- Fats from other sources like beef tallow, avocado, mayonnaise, butter, olive oil, coconut oil, chicken fat, ghee, coconut butter, non-hydrogenated lard, red palm oil, macadamia nuts, and peanut butter.

- Saturated fats like lard, tallow, goose fat, chicken fat, duck fat, clarified butter, and coconut oil

- Monounsaturated fats like avocado, olive oil, and macadamia nuts

- Polyunsaturated fats like fatty fish and other seafood

- For vegetable oils, cold-pressed options like flax, safflower, soybean, and olive oil are recommended

Meats – Focus should be on lean meat, preferably wild caught or organic fed

- Organic eggs and poultry

- Grass-fed meat like goat, venison, lamb, and beef

- Organic pork and derivative products like butter, ghee, and gelatine, but not meat covered in sugary or starchy sauces, and breadcrumbs.

- Wild-caught fish like catfish, cod, mackerel, flounder, halibut, snapper, tuna, mahi-mahi, trout, and salmon

- Wild-caught shellfish and seafood such as squid, shrimps, clams, lobsters, oysters, crabs, mussels, and scallops

- Innards or offal like kidney, heart, liver and other similar organ meats.

Other Food Sources

- Beverages like tea, coffee, and water

- Fresh spices like basil, sea salt, chili powder, black pepper, cinnamon, cayenne powder, cilantro, parsley, oregano, sage, cumin, sage, thyme and turmeric

- Dairy products like heavy whipping cream, hard and soft cheese, cottage cheese, and sour cream

- Seeds and nuts like walnuts, macadamia nuts, almonds, cashews, pistachios, and flour derived from nuts

- Sweeteners like liquid stevia and sucralose, xylitol, erythritol, monk fruit, and small amounts of agave nectar.

What to Avoid

To put it simply, you should avoid all processed, sugary, carbohydrate-rich, and farmed food. Following is a more comprehensive list:

Fruits – In general, fruits should be eaten in moderation, but avoid the ones on this list:

- Tropical fruits like banana, pineapple, papaya, and mango

- Fruits with high carbohydrate content like tangerine and grapes

- Fruit juices; as an alternative you can go for fruits in smoothie form because these have retained the fiber content.

Fats – Although keto encourages fat consumptions, avoid these unhealthy fats:

- Refined oils and fats like canola, sunflower, grapeseed, corn oil, and cottonseed

- Trans fats like margarine

Meat and seafood - Avoid the farmed and processed varieties as they are rich in fatty acids like omega-6 that induce inflammation.

- Root crops like carrots, potatoes, sweet potatoes, turnips, parsnips, beets, and radish

- Grains and grain-derived products like rye, oats, wheat, corn, barley, sorghum, millet, buckwheat, rice, sprouted grains, and amaranth

- Quinoa

- Sweets and sugary food like ice cream, cakes, and sweet pudding

Sweeteners – Avoid artificial sweeteners as they may trigger cravings and various health concerns.

- Sweeteners that contain Acesulfame, Aspartame, Saccharine, and Sucralose

- Equal or Splenda

- Products labelled as zero-carb, low-fat or low-carb like mints and gums, and diet sodas as they may have artificial ingredients.

Dairy Products – Take milk only in moderation.

Beverages – Avoid sodas, sugary drinks, and alcoholic beverages.

Tracking Your Food Intake

When using the ketogenic diet, one key to success is to effectively monitor your food intake or macros.

Following is the ideal ratio of macronutrient calories in the ketogenic diet:

- Fat – 60 to 75%

- Protein – 15 to 30%

- Carbohydrates – 5 to 10%

To make sure that you stay within the recommended limits, it is crucial that you take note of everything you consume while on this diet. The good thing is you can customize the macronutrient ratio to meet your specific needs and preferences. However, you should make sure that your fat consumption remains high, while keeping your carb intake on the low side.

When calculating and setting your macros, you must consider your physical activity level as well as how your body will respond to the ratio. There are many apps today that you can use as aid in calculating and tracking your macros. This way, you will always be updated on how you much fats, protein, and carbs you are consuming on a meal by meal basis.

The apps can also help you discover the kinds of nutrients you are getting and the ones that you need more of. Ultimately, once you have gotten used to the various types of food you need and don't need, you may find no more use in your tracking tools. Thus, even when dining out with family and friends, you will know how to estimate your macro consumption and accordingly portion your meals.

Chapter 2: Breakfast Recipes

GREEN SMOOTHIE KETO BREAKFAST

Prep time: 5 min; **Cook time**: 0 min

Serving Size: 1 glass; **Serves**: 1

Calories: 380; **Total Fat**: 30 g; **Protein**: 12 g;

Total Carbs: 13 g; **Net Carbs**: 5 g; **Sugar**: 0 g; **Fiber**: 8 g;

Ingredients

- 10 pcs. of raw almonds

- 2 cups of kale or spinach

- 2 pcs. of Brazil nuts

- 1 scoop of Amazing Grass Greens Powder or green powder of your choice

- 1 cup of unsweetened coconut milk (from a refrigerated carton and not in can)

Instructions

1. Place the almonds, spinach, coconut milk and Brazil nuts into the blender.

2. Blend the ingredients until pureed.

3. Add the rest of the ingredients.

4. Blend well.

5. Serve in a tall glass and enjoy.

Scrambled Eggs w/ Guacamole Topping

Prep time: 5 min; **Cook time**: 10 min

Serving Size: 1 plate; **Serves**: 1

Calories: 442; **Total Fat**: 23 g; **Protein**: 18 g;

Total Carbs: 4 g; **Net Carbs**: 2 g; **Sugar**: 0 g; **Fiber**: 2 g;

Ingredients

- 3 medium-sized eggs
- 1 Tbsp. of coconut oil
- ¼ cup of guacamole (any brand like Wholly Guacamole)
- 1 pinch of salt, to taste

Instructions

1. Put coconut oil in the pan.
2. Put the eggs, and scramble over low heat setting.
3. Transfer the scrambled eggs into a serving plate.
4. Top eggs with guacamole.
5. Add a pinch of salt, if desired.
6. Serve and enjoy.

Breakfast Bacon Lemon Thyme Muffins

Prep time: 15 min; **Cook time**: 20 min

Serving Size: 2 muffins; **Serves**: 6

Calories: 300; **Total Fat**: 28 g; **Protein**: 11 g;

Total Carbs: 7 g; **Net Carbs**: 4 g; **Sugar**: 1 g; **Fiber**: 3 g;

Ingredients

- 3 cups of almond flour
- 4 medium-sized eggs
- 1 cup of bacon bits
- 2 tsp. of lemon thyme
- ½ cup of melted ghee
- 1 tsp. of baking soda
- ½ tsp. of salt, to taste

Equipment needed

- Muffin pan
- Muffin liners

Instructions

1. Pre-heat oven to 350⁰ F.

2. Put ghee in mixing bowl and melt.

3. Add baking soda and almond flour.

4. Put the eggs in.

5. Add the lemon thyme (if preferred, other herbs or spices may be used).

6. Drizzle with salt.

7. Mix all ingredients well.

8. Sprinkle with bacon bits

9. Line the muffin pan with liners.

10. Spoon mixture into the pan, filling the pan to about ¾ full.

11. Bake for about 20 minutes. Test by inserting a toothpick into a muffin. If it comes out clean, then the muffins are done.

12. Serve immediately.

Bowl of Matcha Smoothie

Prep time: 10 min; **Cook time**: 0 min

Serving Size: 1 bowl; **Serves**: 1

Calories: 420; **Total Fat**: 28 g; **Protein**: 13 g;

Total Carbs: 25 g; **Net Carbs**: 8 g; **Sugar**: 6 g; **Fiber**: 17 g;

Ingredients

- 1 tsp. of matcha powder
- 1 scoop of greens powder (if desired)
- 8 oz. of coconut yogurt (may be substituted w/ regular Greek yogurt if you have no problems with dairy)
- 1 Tbsp. of goji berries
- 1 Tbsp. of chia seeds
- 1 Tbsp. of cacao nibs
- 1 Tbsp. of coconut flakes
- Stevia, to taste

Instructions

1. Blend the yogurt with the matcha powder. Sweeten with stevia, if preferred.

2. Transfer the smoothie into a regular-sized bowl.

3. Top the smoothie with goji berries, chia seeds, cacao nibs, and coconut flakes

4. Serve and enjoy.

SUPER QUICKIE SCRAMBLE

Prep time: 10 min; **Cook time**: 15 min

Serving Size: 1 plate; **Serves**: 1

Calories: 350; **Total Fat**: 29 g; **Protein**: 21 g;

Total Carbs: 5 g; **Net Carbs**: 4 g; **Sugar**: 3 g; **Fiber**: 1 g;

Ingredients

- 3 small sized eggs, whisked
- 4 pcs. bella mushrooms
- ½ cup of spinach
- ¼ cup of red bell peppers
- 2 deli ham slices
- 1 tablespoon of ghee or coconut oil
- Salt & pepper to taste

Instructions

1. Chop the ham and veggies.
2. Put half a tablespoon of butter in a frying pan and heat until melted.

3. Sauté the ham and vegetables in a frying pan then set aside.

4. Get a new frying pan and heat the remaining butter.

5. Add the whisked eggs into the second pan while stirring continuously to avoid overcooking.

6. When the eggs are done, sprinkle with salt & pepper to taste.

7. Add the ham and veggies to the pan with the eggs.

8. Mix well.

9. Remove from heat and transfer to a plate.

10. Serve and enjoy.

Coconut Coffee and Ghee

Prep time: 5 - 10 min; **Cook time**: 0 min

Serving Size: 1 cup; **Serves**: 1

Calories: 150; **Total Fat**: 15 g; **Protein**: 0 g;

Total Carbs: 0 g; **Net Carbs**: 0 g; **Sugar**: 0 g; **Fiber**: 0 g;

Ingredients

- ½ Tbsp. of coconut oil

- ½ Tbsp. of ghee

- 1 to 2 cups of preferred coffee (or rooibos or black tea, if preferred)

- 1 Tbsp. of coconut or almond milk

Instructions

1. Place the almond (or coconut) milk, coconut oil, ghee and coffee in a blender (or milk frother).

2. Process for around 10 seconds or until the coffee turns creamy and foamy.

3. Pour contents into a coffee cup.

4. Serve immediately and enjoy.

Poached Egg w/ Spring Soup

Prep time: 10 min; **Cook time**: 20 min

Serving Size: 1 bowl; **Serves**: 2

Calories: 150; **Total Fat**: 5 g; **Protein**: 16 g;

Total Carbs: 11 g; **Net Carbs**: 4 g; **Sugar**: 5 g; **Fiber**: 7 g;

Ingredients

- 32 oz. of chicken broth
- 2 regular-sized eggs
- 1 head romaine lettuce, chopped
- 1 pinch of salt, to taste

Instructions

1. Boil the chicken broth.
2. Turn the heat down, then poach the eggs in the broth for around 5 minutes or until slightly runny.
3. Get the eggs and transfer into separate bowls.
4. Place the chopped romaine lettuce in the soup, and cook for 3 to 5 minutes or until wilted slightly.
5. Using a ladle, transfer the broth into the 2 bowls.

6. Serve while hot and enjoy immediately.

BRIE BALLS & SALTED CARAMEL

Prep time: 5 min; **Cook time**: 0 min

Serving Size: 1 ball; **Serves**: 6

Calories: 130; **Total Fat**: 12 g; **Protein**: 5 g;

Total Carbs: 1 g; **Net Carbs**: 0 g; **Sugar**: 1 g; **Fiber**: 1 g;

Ingredients

- 4 oz. of Brie cheese, chopped roughly

- 2 oz. of salted macadamia nuts

- ½ tsp. of caramel flavor

Instructions

1. Place all ingredients in a small-sized food processor and pulse until a coarse dough is formed or around half a minute.

2. Using a spoon, form 6 balls from the mixture.

3. Serve and enjoy immediately. If desired, refrigerate for no more than 3 days before consuming.

OLD-FASHIONED STEAK AND EGGS

Prep time: 15 min; **Cook time**: 30 min

Serving Size: 1 plate; **Serves**: 1

Calories: 687; **Total Fat**: 52 g; **Protein**: 43 g;

Total Carbs: 5 g; **Net Carbs**: 5 g; **Sugar**: 0 g; **Fiber**: 0 g;

Ingredients:

- 4 oz. of sirloin steak (or any preferred steak cut)
- 3 large-sized eggs
- 1 Tbsp. of butter
- 1 Tbsp. of olive oil
- ½ avocado
- Salt & pepper to taste

Instructions

1. Heat the olive oil in a pan and cook the steak until the desired doneness is achieved.

2. While waiting for the sirloin to cook, get another pan and heat the butter until it is completely melted. Fry the eggs until the yolks reach the preferred level of doneness

and the egg whites have set. Dash a pinch of salt & pepper.

3. Remove the sirloin steak from the pan and slice it into bite-sized pieces. Season with some salt & pepper.

4. Cut the avocado into smaller slices. Sprinkle with some salt.

5. Assemble everything on a plate.

6. Serve and enjoy immediately.

CARBONARA BALLS

Prep time: 8 min; **Cook time**: 0 min

Serving Size: 1 ball; **Serves**: 6

Calories: 148; **Total Fat**: 12 g; **Protein**: 8 g;

Total Carbs: 1 g; **Net Carbs**: 1 g; **Sugar**: 1 g; **Fiber**: 0 g;

Ingredients

- 3 oz. of bacon, cooked

- 3 oz. mascarpone

- 2 large-sized eggs (hard-boiled, use the yolks only)

- ¼ tsp. black pepper, freshly ground

Instructions

1. Chop the cooked bacon into crumbs.

2. Place the egg yolks, pepper, and mascarpone in a small-sized bowl. Use a fork to mix everything well.

3. Form 6 balls from the mixture.

4. Put the bacon crumbs on a medium-sized plate. Roll the balls through, making sure each ball is evenly coated.

5. Serve and enjoy immediately. If preferred, refrigerate first before serving, and use within 3 days.

Low Carb & Gluten Free Breakfast Casserole ala Monte Cristo

Prep time: 15 min; **Cook time**: 15 min

Serving Size: 3 ½ to 4 in² square; **Serves**: 6

Calories: 376; **Total Fat**: 24 g; **Protein**: 32 g;

Total Carbs: 4.5 g; **Net Carbs**: 4.5 g; **Sugar**: 0 g; **Fiber**: 0 g;

Ingredients

- 3 batches of cream cheese pancakes

- (2) 6-oz packages of bacon

- 1 ½ cups of shredded Swiss or Gruyere cheese

- ½ cup of warmed sugar-free pancake syrup

Instructions

1. Grease a medium-sized baking dish.

2. Put a layer of cream cheese pancakes (4 pcs) at the bottom and around halfway up the sides.

3. Place a layer of bacon, and then sprinkle with half a cup of cheese.

4. Bake for 15 minutes at 375⁰ F or until heated all over.

5. Take the dish out of the oven and then evenly pour warm syrup on top.

6. Cut the dish into six squares

7. Serve and enjoy while warm.

Hot Bacon and Avocado Balls

Prep time: 45 min; **Cook time**: 8 min

Serving Size: 1 ball; **Serves**: 6

Calories: 181; **Total Fat**: 18 g; **Protein**: 3 g;

Total Carbs: 3 g; **Net Carbs**: 1 g; **Sugar**: 0 g; **Fiber**: 2 g;

Ingredients

- 4 slices of bacon

- 1 medium-sized avocado, pitted & peeled

- 1 Tbsp. of bacon fat

- 1 Tbsp. of green onions, chopped finely

- 2 Tbsp. of cilantro, chopped finely

- 1 small-sized jalapeño pepper, seeded & chopped finely

- 2 Tbsp. of coconut oil

- 1/3 tsp. of sea salt

Instructions

1. Put a non-stick skillet over heat set at medium. Cook the bacon slices until they turn golden. This should take around 4 minutes for each side.

2. Drain the excess oil from the bacon using a paper towel. Set the bacon fat aside in a glass container. Allow the bacon to cool.

3. Chop two of the bacon slices into crumbs.

4. Cut the remaining 2 slices of bacon into 3 pieces each. Set them aside for later. They will serve as the bases of the balls.

5. Using a fork, mash the avocado in a small sized bowl. Pour the cooled bacon fat and coconut oil. Add the onion, jalapeño, cilantro, salt, and bacon crumbles. Mix all the ingredients well.

6. Refrigerate for half an hour, at least.

7. Remove the mixture from the refrigerator.

8. Spoon out the mixture and make 6 balls.

9. Arrange the bacon pieces previously set aside on a plate. Put one avocado ball on top of each piece of bacon.

10. Serve immediately and enjoy. If preferred, refrigerate for no more than 3 days before consuming.

BACON JALAPEÑO BALLS

Prep time: 10 min; **Cook time**: 0 min

Serving Size: 1 ball; **Serves**: 6

Calories: 135; **Total Fat**: 11 g; **Protein**: 7 g;

Total Carbs: 1 g; **Net Carbs**: 1 g; **Sugar**: 0 g; **Fiber**: 0 g;

Ingredients

- 3 oz. of cooked bacon (reserve the fat)
- 3 oz. of cream cheese
- 1 Tbsp. of cilantro, chopped finely
- 2 Tbsp. of reserved bacon fat
- 1 tsp. of jalapeño pepper, seeded & chopped finely

Instructions

1. Get a cutting board and chop the cooked bacon into bits.

2. Get a small-sized bowl and mix the jalapeño, cream cheese, cilantro, and bacon fat well. From the mixture, form 6 balls.

3. On a medium-sized plate, spread out the bacon crumbs. Individually roll the balls, making sure that each one is coated evenly.

4. Serve and enjoy immediately. If preferred, refrigerate first before serving, and use within 3 days.

SALAMI & OLIVE ROLLUPS

Prep time: 5 min; **Cook time**: 0 min

Serving Size: 1 wrap; **Serves**: 3

Calories: 233; **Total Fat**: 20 g; **Protein**: 8 g;

Total Carbs: 6 g; **Net Carbs**: 6 g; **Sugar**: 1 g; **Fiber**: 0 g;

Ingredients

- 3 oz. of cream cheese

- 12 pcs. of large, pitted kalamata olives

- 1 (1 oz.) slices of Italian salami

Instructions:

1. Place the cream cheese and olives in a small-sized food processor, and process until a coarse dough consistency is achieved.

2. Using a spoon, form 3 balls from the cheese mixture.

3. Put a ball each on the salami slices. Wrap each ball with a salami, secured by a toothpick.

4. Serve and enjoy immediately. If preferred, refrigerate first before serving, and use within 3 days.

Egg, Sausage, & Cheese

Prep time: 10 min; **Cook time**: 10 min

Serving Size: 1 plate; **Serves**: 1

Calories: 574; **Total Fat**: 49 g; **Protein**: 27 g;

Total Carbs: 1 g; **Net Carbs**: 1 g; **Sugar**: 0 g; **Fiber**: 0 g;

Ingredients

- 3 oz. of breakfast sausage
- 1 large-sized egg
- 1 slice of cheddar cheese
- 1 Tbsp. of olive oil
- Chives or green onion for garnish

Instructions

1. Heat olive oil in a pan, and cook the egg (over easy) and breakfast sausage.
2. Remove from heat and transfer to a plate
3. Add a cheddar slice.
4. Arrange or layer the rest of the ingredients as desired.

5. If preferred, sprinkle some hot sauce.

6. Top everything with sliced green onions or chives.

7. Serve and enjoy immediately.

Chapter 3: Lunch Recipes

TAMARI MARINATED STEAK SALAD

Prep time: 10 min; **Cook time**: 15 min

Serving Size: 1 plate; **Serves**: 2

Calories: 500; **Total Fat**: 37 g; **Protein**: 33 g;

Total Carbs: 4 g; **Net Carbs**: 2 g; **Sugar**: 1 g; **Fiber**: 2 g;

Ingredients

- 2.5 oz. of salad greens
- 6 to 8 pcs. of cherry or grape tomatoes, halved
- ½ pc. of red bell pepper, sliced
- 4 pcs. of radish, sliced
- 1 Tbsp. of olive oil
- ½ Tbsp. of fresh lemon juice
- Salt, to taste
- ½ lb. of steak
- ¼ cup of tamari soy sauce (gluten-free)
- Avocado or olive oil for cooking the steak

Instructions

1. Marinade steak in gluten-free tamari soy sauce.

2. Get a mixing bowl.

3. Start preparing the salad by mixing the tomatoes, bell pepper, salad greens, and radishes with the lemon juice and olive oil. Sprinkle some salt, to taste.

4. Divide and transfer the salad into 2 plates.

5. Put avocado oil (or olive oil) in the frying pan. Set heat on high setting.

6. Cook (or grill) the marinated steak to the preferred doneness level.

7. Transfer the steak into a platter. Set aside for a minute.

8. Slice the steak into strips, and distribute evenly on top of the 2 plates of salad.

Chicken Bites Wrapped in Garlic Bacon

Prep time: 15 min; **Cook time**: 30 min

Serving Size: 1; **Serves**: 4

Calories: 230; **Total Fat**: 13 g; **Protein**: 22 g;

Total Carbs: 5 g; **Net Carbs**: 4 g; **Sugar**: 2 g; **Fiber**: 1 g;

Ingredients

- 1 large-sized chicken breast, cut into around 25 bite-sized pieces

- 8 to 9 thin bacon slices, cut into 3 pcs. each

- 6 pcs. of crushed garlic or 3 Tbsp. of garlic powder

Instructions

1. Pre-heat oven to 400^0 F.

2. Get a baking tray and line with aluminium foil.

3. Put crushed garlic or garlic powder in a mixing bowl

4. Dip each bite-sized chicken piece in garlic.

5. Wrap each piece of chicken with a short piece of bacon.

6. Arrange the bacon-wrapped chicken on the tray. Make sure to have enough space between each chicken piece on the baking tray so they will not touch one another.

7. Place the tray in the oven and bake for 25 to 30 minutes. If possible, turn the chicken pieces after 15 minutes.

SARDINES MUSTARD SALAD

Prep time: 10 min; **Cook time**: 0 min

Serving Size: 1 plate; **Serves**: 1

Calories: 260; **Total Fat**: 20 g; **Protein**: 25 g;

Total Carbs: 0 g; **Net Carbs**: 0 g; **Sugar**: 0 g; **Fiber**: 0 g;

Ingredients

- 4 to 5 oz. (1 can) of sardines in olive oil
- ¼ pc. of cucumber, peeled and cut into small dice
- 1 Tbsp. of lemon juice
- ½ Tbsp. of mustard
- Salt & pepper, to taste

Instructions

1. Drain the sardines of excess olive oil.
2. Mash the sardines.
3. Mix the sardines, lemon juice, diced cucumber, mustard and salt & pepper. Make sure the ingredients are well-combined.
4. Transfer the ingredients to a serving dish and serve.

Chicken Noodle Soup

Prep time: 15 min; **Cook time**: 25 min

Serving Size: 1 bowl; **Serves**: 2

Calories: 310; **Total Fat**: 16 g; **Protein**: 34 g;

Total Carbs: 6 g; **Net Carbs**: 4 g; **Sugar**: 3 g; **Fiber**: 2 g;

Ingredients

- 3 cups of chicken broth
- 1 pc. of chicken breast (around ½ lb.), cut into small pcs.
- 1 pc. of green onion, sliced or chopped
- 1 stalk of celery, sliced or chopped
- 1 pc. of zucchini, peeled
- ¼ cup of cilantro, chopped finely
- Salt, to taste

Instructions

1. Dice the chicken breast.
2. Heat a saucepan with avocado oil.
3. Sauté the chicken pieces until cooked.

4. Add the chicken broth to the diced chicken, and simmer.

5. Add the chopped celery into the saucepan.

6. Add the chopped green onions into the saucepan.

7. Prepare the zucchini noodles. You can use a potato peeler to make long strands or use other methods such as using a food processor (w/ shredding attachment) or spiralizer.

8. Add the zucchini noodles and the chopped cilantro into the pot.

9. Allow to simmer for a few more minutes. Dash with a pinch of salt to taste.

10. Transfer to a bowl and serve while hot. Enjoy!

BABY ZUCCHINI AVOCADO BURGERS

Prep time: 20 min; **Cook time**: 20 min

Serving Size: 1 plate; **Serves**: 2

Calories: 370; **Total Fat**: 30 g; **Protein**: 23 g;

Total Carbs: 9 g; **Net Carbs**: 3 g; **Sugar**: 4 g; **Fiber**: 6 g;

Ingredients

- 1 pc. large-sized zucchini, chopped into ½" slices (makes around 14 to 16 slices)

- ½ lb. of ground beef

- ¼ avocado sliced into small pieces

- 2 Tbsp. avocado or olive oil for greasing the baking tray

- 2 tsp. of salt

- 1 Tbsp. of mustard

- 1 Tbsp. of Greek yogurt (store-bought)

Instructions

1. Preheat the oven to 400⁰ F.

2. Grease the baking tray with avocado oil; sprinkle 1 tsp. of salt across the tray.

3. Put the slices of zucchini into the tray.

4. Make small balls out of the ground beef then press them into patties. You should be able to form 7 to 8 patties. Put the patties on the tray.

5. Put the baking tray in the oven and bake for around 15 minutes. If preferred, you can pan-fry the beef patties and zucchini in avocado oil or grill them, instead of baking.

6. Thinly slice the avocado into small pieces.

7. Using the zucchini slices as burger buns, assemble the baby/mini burgers. Place an avocado slice on each burger, then top with mustard and Greek yogurt.

BROCCOLI BACON SALAD W/ COCONUT CREAM & ONIONS

Prep time: 10 min; **Cook time**: 20 min

Serving Size: 1 bowl; **Serves**: 6

Calories: 280; **Total Fat**: 26 g; **Protein**: 7 g;

Total Carbs: 8 g; **Net Carbs**: 5 g; **Sugar**: 2 g; **Fiber**: 3 g;

Ingredients

- 1 lb. of broccoli florets

- 2 pcs. of large-sized or 4 pcs. of small-sized red onions, sliced

- 1 cup of coconut cream

- 20 bacon slices, cut into small pieces

- Salt, to taste

Instructions

1. Fry the bacon. Using the bacon fat, cook the onions.

2. Blanche the broccoli florets. If preferred, instead of blanching, you can boil them to soften or use them raw.

3. Toss the bacon, broccoli florets, and onions with the coconut cream. Dash with salt to taste.

4. Best served and consumed at room temperature.

Easy Sauté Zucchini Beef w/ Cilantro & Garlic

Prep time: 10 min; **Cook time**: 20 min

Serving Size: 300 g; **Serves**: 2

Calories: 500; **Total Fat**: 40 g; **Protein**: 31 g;

Total Carbs: 5 g; **Net Carbs**: 4 g; **Sugar**: 2 g; **Fiber**: 1 g;

Ingredients

- 10 oz. of beef, sliced against the grain (if possible) into 1 to 2" strips

- 1 pc. of zucchini, sliced thinly into 1 to 2" long strips

- 3 cloves of garlic, minced or diced

- ¼ cup of cilantro, chopped

- Avocado oil for cooking (olive or coconut oil, if preferred)

- 2 Tbsp. gluten-free tamari sauce

Instructions

1. Heat 2 Tbsp. of avocado oil on high heat setting.

2. Put the beef strips into the pan. Sauté on high heat for a couple of minutes.

3. Once the beef browns, toss the zucchini strips in, and continue to sauté.

4. When the zucchini softens, add the garlic, cilantro, and tamari sauce.

5. Saute for a few more minutes.

6. Remove from heat and transfer into a plate.

7. Serve immediately.

TUNA AVOCADO SALAD

Prep time: 10 min; **Cook time**: 0 min

Serving Size: 1 bowl; **Serves**: 1

Calories: 508; **Total Fat**: 34 g; **Protein**: 31 g;

Total Carbs: 5 g; **Net Carbs**: 5 g; **Sugar**: 0 g; **Fiber**: 0 g;

Ingredients

- 4 oz. tuna (canned)
- 1 medium-sized egg, hard-boiled, peeled, & chopped
- ½ pc. of avocado
- ½ stalk of celery, diced
- 2 Tbsp. of mayonnaise
- ½ tsp. of fresh lemon juice
- 1 tsp. of mustard
- Salt & pepper to taste

Instructions

1. In a small-sized bowl, mix the tuna, celery, and avocado.

2. Stir in the mayonnaise, lemon juice, mustard, and spices and then add the chopped egg.

3. Mix everything well.

4. Serve and enjoy immediately, or if preferred, allow to cool in the refrigerator for up to an hour first.

CURRIED TUNA BALLS

Prep time: 10 min; **Cook time**: 0 min

Serving Size: 1 ball; **Serves**: 6

Calories: 93; **Total Fat**: 8 g; **Protein**: 5 g;

Total Carbs: 1 g; **Net Carbs**: 0 g; **Sugar**: 1 g; **Fiber**: 0 g;

Ingredients

- 3 oz. of tuna in oil, drained

- 1 oz. of crumbled macadamia nuts

- 2 oz. of cream cheese

- ¼ tsp. of curry powder, divided

Instructions:

1. Process the tuna, half of the curry powder, and cream cheese in a small-sized food processor. It should take about half a minute before the desired smooth and creamy consistency is achieved.

2. Form 6 balls from the mixture.

3. Place the remaining curry powder and crumbled macadamia nuts on a medium-sized plate.

4. Roll the balls individually to make sure each one is evenly coated.

5. Serve and enjoy immediately. If preferred, refrigerate first before serving, and use within 3 days.

CHICKEN SKIN CRISPS WITH AIOLI EGG SALAD

Prep time: 5 min; **Cook time**: 20 min

Serving Size: 1 bowl; **Serves**: 6

Calories: 79; **Total Fat**: 5 g; **Protein**: 8 g;

Total Carbs: 0 g; **Net Carbs**: 0 g; **Sugar**: 0 g; **Fiber**: 0 g;

Ingredients

- Skin from 3 to 4 pcs. of chicken thighs
- 1 large-sized hardboiled egg, yolk only, chopped
- 1 large-sized hardboiled egg, peeled & chopped
- 1 Tbsp. of fresh parsley, chopped finely
- 1 Tbsp. of mayonnaise
- ¼ pc. of garlic clove, minced
- ½ tsp. of sea salt

Instructions

1. Set oven to 350⁰ F and preheat.

2. Lay out the skins on a cookie sheet. Make sure they are as flat as possible.

3. Allow to bake for 12 to 15 minutes or until the skins become crispy and light brownish. Make sure they don't burn.

4. Take the skins from the cookie sheet and transfer to a paper towel. Allow to cool for a few minutes.

5. Combine the egg yolk, egg, mayonnaise, garlic, sea salt, and parsley in a small-sized bowl and mix well.

6. Halve each piece of crispy chicken skin.

7. Put a Tbsp. of the egg salad mixture on top of each chicken crisp.

8. Serve and enjoy right away.

SHRIMP WITH GARLIC SAUCE

Prep time: 5 min; **Cook time**: 5 min

Serving Size: 1 plate; **Serves**: 2

Calories: 335; **Total Fat**: 27 g; **Protein**: 22 g;

Total Carbs: 2.5 g; **Net Carbs**: 2.5 g; **Sugar**: 0 g; **Fiber**: 0 g;

Ingredients

- ½ lb. of large shrimp

- 2 cloves of garlic, minced

- ¼ tsp. of cayenne

- ¼ cup of olive oil

- 1 wedge of lemon

- Salt & pepper to taste

Instructions

1. Pour some olive oil in a small-sized pan. Set heat to medium-low. Add the cayenne and garlic, and cook until the fragrance pervades the air.

2. Peel the shrimp and devein as necessary. Cook each side for 2 to 3 minutes.

3. Drizzle with salt & pepper. Squeeze the lemon wedge on the shrimp.

4. The dish is best served warm. You can use the remaining garlic oil as dipping sauce served separate from the dish.

CHICKEN SKIN CRISPS SATAY

Prep time: 5 min; **Cook time**: 20 min

Serving Size: 1 plate; **Serves**: 6

Calories: 91; **Total Fat**: 5 g; **Protein**: 8 g;

Total Carbs: 3 g; **Net Carbs**: 3 g; **Sugar**: 2 g; **Fiber**: 0 g;

Ingredients:

- Skin from 3 to 4 pcs. of chicken thighs
- 2 Tbsp. of chunky peanut butter
- 1 Tbsp. of coconut cream
- 1 tsp. of coconut oil
- 1 tsp. of jalapeño pepper, fresh, seeded & minced
- 1 tsp. of coconut aminos
- ¼ clove of garlic, minced

Instructions

1. Pre-heat oven to 350⁰ F.
2. Lay out the skins on a cookie sheet. Make sure they are as flat as possible.

3. Bake the skins for 12 to 15 minutes or until they become crispy and light brown. Make sure they don't burn.

4. Take the skins from the cookie sheet and transfer to a paper towel. Allow to cool for a few minutes.

5. Put the peanut butter, jalapeños, coconut oil, coconut aminos, and garlic in a small-sized food processor. Process until everything is well-blended or for around 30 seconds.

6. Cut the crispy chicken skins into 2 pieces. Make sure each one is approximately of the same size.

7. Put a Tbsp. of peanut sauce on top of each piece of chicken crisp.

8. Serve and enjoy immediately. However, if you find the sauce a bit runny, you can refrigerate it first for up to two hours before you use it.

Chicken Skin Crisps Alfredo

Prep time: 5 min; **Cook time**: 20 min

Serving Size: 1; **Serves**: 6

Calories: 71; **Total Fat**: 4 g; **Protein**: 8 g;

Total Carbs: 1 g; **Net Carbs**: 1 g; **Sugar**: 0 g; **Fiber**: 0 g;

Ingredients

- Skin from 3 to 4 pcs. of chicken thighs
- 2 Tbsp. of cream cheese
- 2 Tbsp. of ricotta
- 1 Tbsp. of Parmesan cheese, grated
- ¼ pc. of garlic clove, minced
- ¼ tsp. of white pepper, ground

Instructions

1. Pre-heat oven to 350⁰ F.
2. Lay out the skins on a cookie sheet. Make sure they are as flat as possible.
3. Bake the skins for 12 to 15 minutes or until they become crispy and light brown. Make sure they don't burn.

4. Take the skins from the cookie sheet and transfer to a paper towel. Allow to cool for a few minutes.

5. Get a small-sized bowl and mix the pepper, garlic and cheeses. Mix everything until well-blended.

6. Cut the crispy chicken skins into 2 pieces. Make sure each one is approximately of the same size.

7. Put a Tbsp. of the Alfredo cheese mix on top of the chicken crisps.

8. Serve and enjoy immediately.

MEDITERRANEAN ROLLUPS

Prep time: 7 min; **Cook time**: 3 min

Serving Size: 1 frittata; **Serves**: 2

Calories: 153; **Total Fat**: 10 g; **Protein**: 5 g;

Total Carbs: 14 g; **Net Carbs**: 12 g; **Sugar**: 5 g; **Fiber**: 2 g;

Ingredients

- 1 pc. of large-sized egg

- 6 pcs of large-sized kalamata olives, pitted

- 1 oz. of sun-dried tomatoes in oil

- 1 Tbsp. of extra virgin olive oil

- 1/8 tsp. of sea salt

- 1/8 tsp. of parsley flakes

- 1/8 tsp. of red chili flakes

Instructions

1. Combine the olive oil, salt and egg in a small-sized bowl. Whisk until a foamy consistency is achieved.

2. Heat a small-sized non-stick pan over high setting. Pour the egg mixture in, spreading evenly and thinly.

3. Cook one side first for about one minute before flipping the frittata. Cook the other side until the bottom turns golden. This will take about 2 minutes more.

4. Remove from heat and transfer to a plate.

5. Combine the chili flakes, olives, parsley, and tomatoes in a small-sized food processor. Process until everything is chopped and blended well or around 30 seconds.

6. Top the frittata with an even layer of olive paste.

7. Roll the frittata tightly.

8. Cut the roll in 2 pieces.

9. Serve and enjoy immediately.

Smoked Salmon and Crème Fraîche Rollups

Prep time: 5 min; **Cook time**: 0 min

Serving Size: 1 roll; **Serves**: 3

Calories: 87; **Total Fat**: 7 g; **Protein**: 6 g;

Total Carbs: 8 g; **Net Carbs**: 8 g; **Sugar**: 1 g; **Fiber**: 0 g;

Ingredients

- 3 oz. of crème Fraîche (or French sour cream)
- 1/8 tsp. of fresh lemon zest
- 3 slices of smoked salmon or lox
- 1/8 teaspoon fresh lemon zest
- 3 slices (1 oz.) of smoked salmon (lox)

Instructions

1. Mix the French sour cream and lemon zest in a small-sized bowl.

2. Evenly top each slice of salmon with of the mixture.

3. Individually roll each slice, and secure the rolls with toothpicks.

4. Serve and enjoy immediately.

Chapter 4: Dinner Recipes

THAI CHICKEN & RICE

Prep time: 15 min; **Cook time**: 30 min

Serving Size: 1 large bowl; **Serves**: 4

Calories: 350; **Total Fat**: 11 g; **Protein**: 55 g;

Total Carbs: 9 g; **Net Carbs**: 5 g; **Sugar**: 4 g; **Fiber**: 4 g;

Ingredients

- 1 pc. of cauliflower head
- 3 to 4 pcs. of cooked chicken breasts or meat from 1 whole chicken, shredded
- 3 medium-sized eggs
- 3 pcs. of chilies (any preferred variety will do)
- 1 Tbsp. of ginger, freshly grated
- 3 cloves of regular-sized garlic, crushed
- Coconut oil for cooking
- Salt to taste
- 1 Tbsp. of tamari soy sauce or coconut aminos (optional)
- ½ cup of cilantro, chopped (for garnishing)

Instructions

1. Separate the cauliflower into florets, then process in a food processor until a rice-like texture is achieved. It may be done in several batches, if necessary.

2. Get a large pan and cook the processed cauliflower in coconut oil. If necessary, do it in batches or in 2 separate pans. Set the heat to medium and continue to stir.

3. In a new pan, heat some coconut oil, then scramble the eggs.

4. Combine the scrambled eggs with the rice-like cauliflower.

5. Add the chopped chilies, garlic, and ginger.

6. Once the cauliflower rice softens, gently mix the shredded chicken meat in.

7. Add the tamari soy sauce or coconut aminos to the mix. Sprinkle some salt to taste. Mix everything well.

8. Transfer the dish to a large bowl and garnish with cilantro.

9. Serve immediately; best consumed when hot.

GHEE GARLIC PAN-FRIED COD

Prep time: 10 min; **Cook time**: 15 min

Serving Size: 1 plate; **Serves**: 4

Calories: 160; **Total Fat**: 7 g; **Protein**: 21 g;

Total Carbs: 1 g; **Net Carbs**: 0 g; **Sugar**: 0 g; **Fiber**: 0 g;

Ingredients

- 4 pcs of 0.3-lb. cod fillets

- 6 garlic cloves, minced

- 3 Tbsp. of ghee

- 1 Tbsp. of garlic powder (if preferred)

- Salt, to taste

Instructions

1. Melt ghee in the frying pan.

2. Get half of the minced garlic and toss into the pan.

3. Cook the cod fillets on high to medium setting, then sprinkle with garlic powder and salt.

4. As the cod is cooking, you will notice it turn slowly into a solid white color from being translucent. Wait until the

white color has crept halfway up to the side of the cod fillet. Once it does, flip the fish, and toss in the minced garlic.

5. Continue to cook until the entire file has turned into a solid white color. You will know that the fish is done when it easily flakes.

6. Transfer the fish to a serving dish. Garnish with some ghee and garlic from the frying pan.

7. Serve and enjoy while hot.

Cauliflower Tabbouleh Salad

Prep time: 15 min; **Cook time**: 0 min

Serving Size: 90 g; **Serves**: 2

Calories: 80; **Total Fat**: 7 g; **Protein**: 1 g;

Total Carbs: 5 g; **Net Carbs**: 3 g; **Sugar**: 2 g; **Fiber**: 2 g;

Ingredients

- 100 g of cauliflower florets

- 3 pcs. of mint leaves, diced finely

- 2 Tbsp. of parsley, diced finely

- 2 pcs. of regular-sized tomatoes, diced

- 1 Tbsp. of olive oil

- 1 slice of lemon, diced

- Salt & pepper, to taste

Instructions

1. Process the cauliflower florets in a food processor or blender until a couscous-like texture is achieved. Be sure that both the food processor and the florets are dry to

avoid forming a mash, instead of the desired consistency.

2. Combine the processed florets with the diced tomatoes, herbs, olive oil, and lemon slice. Drizzle with some salt & pepper to taste.

3. Divide the salad into 2 bowls.

4. Serve and enjoy!

BISTEK AND ONIONS

Prep time: 5 min; **Cook time**: 15 min

Serving Size: 1 plate; **Serves**: 4

Calories: 400; **Total Fat**: 30 g; **Protein**: 25 g;

Total Carbs: 10 g; **Net Carbs**: 6 g; **Sugar**: 2 g; **Fiber**: 4 g;

Ingredients

- 4 pcs. of beef cube steaks
- 2 pcs. of medium-sized white onions, sliced thinly
- 1 Tbsp. of pork lard
- 1 ¼ Tbsp. of adobo seasoning (store-bought)
- 1 ½ Tbsp. of coconut vinegar
- 1 Tbsp. of olive oil

Instructions

1. Heat olive oil at medium-high setting then add the onions. Stir frequently until browned. Turn down the heat to medium.

2. Take the cube steaks and dust each side with 1 Tbsp. of adobo seasoning. Once done, sprinkle each side with 1 Tbsp. coconut vinegar. Set aside.

3. Add remaining ¼ Tbsp. of adobo seasoning and ½ Tbsp. of coconut vinegar to the pan. Stir. Create a hole in the heap of onions. Put the cube steaks in the hole. Cover the steaks with onions. Make sure that the beef is directly in contact with the pan.

4. Once the beef begins to brown at the edges, flip using a fork. See to it that there is not too much onions beneath the meat. Allow to cook uncovered until the meat is cooked through. This should only take a few minutes.

5. Transfer the beef steaks and onions to a serving dish.

6. Enjoy while hot.

Thai Chicken & Rice

Prep time: 15 min; **Cook time**: 30 min

Serving Size: 1 large bowl; **Serves**: 4

Calories: 350; **Total Fat**: 11 g; **Protein**: 55 g;

Total Carbs: 9 g; **Net Carbs**: 5 g; **Sugar**: 4 g; **Fiber**: 4 g;

Ingredients

- 1 pc. of cauliflower head
- 3 to 4 pcs. of cooked chicken breasts or meat from 1 whole chicken, shredded
- 3 medium-sized eggs
- 3 pcs. of chilies (any preferred variety will do)
- 1 Tbsp. of ginger, freshly grated
- 3 cloves of regular-sized garlic, crushed
- Coconut oil for cooking
- Salt to taste
- 1 Tbsp. of tamari soy sauce or coconut aminos (optional)
- ½ cup of cilantro, chopped (for garnishing)

Instructions

10. Separate the cauliflower into florets, then process in a food processor until a rice-like texture is achieved. It may be done in several batches, if necessary.

11. Get a large pan and cook the processed cauliflower in coconut oil. If necessary, do it in batches or in 2 separate pans. Set the heat to medium and continue to stir.

12. In a new pan, heat some coconut oil, then scramble the eggs.

13. Combine the scrambled eggs with the rice-like cauliflower.

14. Add the chopped chilies, garlic, and ginger.

15. Once the cauliflower rice softens, gently mix the shredded chicken meat in.

16. Add the tamari soy sauce or coconut aminos to the mix. Sprinkle some salt to taste. Mix everything well.

17. Transfer the dish to a large bowl and garnish with cilantro.

18. Serve immediately; best consumed when hot.

Pork Tenderloin Pan-Fry

Prep time: 10 min; **Cook time**: 25 min

Serving Size: 1 plate; **Serves**: 2

Calories: 330; **Total Fat**: 15 g; **Protein**: 47 g;

Total Carbs: 0 g; **Net Carbs**: 0 g; **Sugar**: 0 g; **Fiber**: 0 g;

Ingredients

- 1 lb. of pork tenderloin

- 1 Tbsp. of coconut oil

- Salt & pepper to taste

Instructions

1. Cut to pork into 2 shorter halves of equal size.

2. Heat a Tbsp. of coconut oil in a frying pan on medium heat setting.

3. Once the coconut oil is completely melted, put the 2 tenderloin halves in the pan.

4. Allow the meat to cook on one side. Once the side is done, use a tong to turn the pork to cook on another side. Just continue to turn and cook until the meat is done on all the sides.

5. The pork is cooked once the meat thermometer displays an internal temperature under 145⁰ F.

6. Take the meat out of the frying pan. You will notice that the pork will still keep on cooking for a little bit more after removing it from the heat.

7. Allow the meat to sit for several minutes before slicing into 1" slices using a sharp knife.

8. Arrange in a serving dish.

9. Serve and enjoy immediately.

Stir-Fried Spinach Almond

Prep time: 5 min; **Cook time**: 20 min

Serving Size: 1 cup; **Serves**: 2

Calories: 150; **Total Fat**: 11 g; **Protein**: 8 g;

Total Carbs: 10 g; **Net Carbs**: 4 g; **Sugar**: 1 g; **Fiber**: 6 g;

Ingredients

- 1 lb. of spinach leaves

- 3 Tbsp. of almond slices

- 1 Tbsp. of coconut oil to cook with

- Salt to taste

Instructions

1. Heat the 1 Tbsp. of coconut oil in a large-sized pot on medium heat setting.

2. Put in the spinach and allow it to cook down a bit.

3. When the spinach has cooked down, sprinkle some salt to taste. Stir

4. Stir the almond slices in.

5. Transfer the contents into a cup.

6. Serve and enjoy.

Skewered Grilled Chicken w/ Garlic Sauce

Prep time: 15 min; **Cook time**: 30 min

Serving Size: 1 large-sized plate; **Serves**: 2

Calories: 580; **Total Fat**: 33 g; **Protein**: 55 g;

Total Carbs: 11 g; **Net Carbs**: 9 g; **Sugar**: 1 g; **Fiber**: 2 g;

Ingredients

For the Skewers

- 1 lb. of chicken breast, cut into 1"-sized cubes

- 2 pcs. of bell peppers, chopped

- 1 pc. of zucchini

- 1 pc. of onion, chopped

For the Garlic Sauce

- 1 pc. of garlic head, peeled

- ¼ cup of lemon juice

- 1 tsp. of salt

- 1 cup of olive oil

For the Marinade

- 1 tsp. of salt

- ½ cup of olive oil

Instructions

1. Start up the grill and set it to high. When using wooden skewers, make sure to soak them first in water.

2. To prepare the garlic sauce, mix the garlic cloves with salt, and process in a blender. Add about ½ cup of the olive oil and 1/8 cup of the lemon juice.

3. Blend everything for around 10 seconds before slowing the blender down. Alternately drizzle some olive oil and lemon juice. Stop only once you hear a subtle sound shift in the blender. By then, you should notice the sauce achieving a mayo-like consistency. In case this does not happen, do not worry. Although your sauce may not look great, it will still have the desired taste.**

4. Set aside ½ of the garlic sauce which will be used when serving the finished dish. Take the rest of the sauce and mix with a tsp. of salt and half a cup of olive oil. Make sure to mix well. This will be your marinade.

5. Mix the chopped chicken, bell peppers, onion, and zucchini in a mixing bowl with the prepared marinade.

6. Put the cubed ingredients on skewers. Put the grill on high heat setting and grill the skewers until the chicken is done. To achieve a charred look grill on the bottom first for a couple of minutes before moving the skewers to a higher rack while the lid is closed to make sure that the chicken is cooked well.

7. Remove from heat and serve with the garlic sauce you previously set aside.

8. Enjoy hot.

** Here's a useful tip to keep in mind: If you have no experience in getting an emulsion or achieving the mayo-like consistency when preparing the sauce, do not get discouraged if you are not successful initially. With practice, you will eventually get it. At first, your sauce may not look delicious, but it is alright because it will still have the same good taste and flavor.

CREAMY CHICKEN TOMATO BASIL PASTA

Prep time: 15 min; **Cook time**: 30 min

Serving Size: 1 large-sized plate; **Serves**: 2

Calories: 540; **Total Fat**: 27 g; **Protein**: 59 g;

Total Carbs: 15 g; **Net Carbs**: 11 g; **Sugar**: 8 g; **Fiber**: 4 g;

Ingredients

- 2 pcs. of chicken breasts, cubed

- 1 can (14 oz. or 400 g) of diced tomatoes

- ½ cup of basil, chopped

- 6 cloves of garlic, minced

- 1 pc. of zucchini, spiralized or shredded for the pasta (as an alternative, spaghetti squash may be used.)

- ¼ cup of coconut milk

- 2 Tbsp. of coconut oil or ghee for use in cooking the dish

- Salt to taste

Instructions

1. Saute the diced meat in coconut oil or ghee until the chicken is slightly browned and cooked.

2. Put the diced tomatoes in, and then sprinkle some salt to taste. Allow the dish to simmer and wait for the liquid to cook down.

3. Meanwhile, you can prepare the pasta. If you are using zucchini, use a spiralizer or julienne peeler to shred it, or if preferred, you can use a food processor. On the other hand, if you want to use spaghetti squash, halve it then take the seeds away. Lightly cover with coconut oil, then microwave the halves for around 7 minutes each.

4. Add the garlic, coconut milk, and basil to the chicken meat and allow to cook for around 5 minutes more.

5. Get 2 bowls and divide the pasta equally into two. Top each bowl with the creamy chicken tomato basil sauce.

6. Serve and enjoy immediately.

Slow Cooked Lemon Rosemary Chicken

Prep time: 15 min; **Cook time**: 30 min

Serving Size: 1; **Serves**:

Calories: 589; **Total Fat**: 40 g; **Protein**: 47 g;

Total Carbs: 4 g; **Net Carbs**: 4 g; **Sugar**: 0 g; **Fiber**: 0 g;

Ingredients

- 3 pcs. of chicken thighs, skinless & boneless
- 1 ½ tsp. of olive oil
- 1 ½ tsp. of garlic, minced
- 1 pc. of lemon
- ¾ tsp. of dried rosemary
- 1 tsp. of thyme, fresh
- ½ tsp. of dried sage, ground
- 1 tsp. of kosher salt

Instructions

1. Put ½ tsp. of salt and garlic in a mortar. Use a pestle to grind and create a paste.

2. Add oil gradually. Grind and mix the paste until it becomes an aioli.

3. Dry off the chicken and put it in a bag together with the aioli. Make sure the chicken is well coated.

4. Marinate the thighs for 2 to 10 hours (marinate longer for better results.)

5. Pre-heat the oven to 425^0 F.

6. Slice the lemon thinly then place the slices at the bottom of the baking pan.

7. Put the thighs on the lemons.

8. Remove the thyme stems and mix the leaves with pepper, sage, rosemary, and what is left of the salt with the chicken.

9. Bake until the juices become clear or around 25 – 30 minutes.

10. Take the chicken out of the pan. Pour the pan drippings into a saucepan.

11. Allow the sauce to boil, while stirring constantly.

12. Lower the heat to medium low. Continue stirring until the sauce reduces.

13. Spoon the sauce generously over the chicken.

14. Immediately serve. Enjoy!

Sunflower Butter Salmon w/ Onions

Prep time: 10 min; **Cook time**: 35 min

Serving Size: 1 plate; **Serves**: 2

Calories: 490; **Total Fat**: 31 g; **Protein**: 44 g;

Total Carbs: 6 g; **Net Carbs**: 6 g; **Sugar**: 0 g; **Fiber**: 0 g;

Ingredients

- 4 oz. of salmon fillet
- 1 to 2 Tbsp. of olive oil
- ½ pc. of onion, sliced
- ¼ tsp. of lemon juice
- ¼ tsp. lemon juice
- 1 Tbsp. of sunflower seed butter
- ½ cup of broccoli, spinach or your preferred low-carb veggie

Instructions

1. Grill the fillet until the desired texture is achieved.
2. In a hot skillet, cook the onions in olive oil until caramelized and color turns to golden-brown.

3. Transfer the onions into a plate.

4. Combine the lemon juice with sunflower seed butter. Heat the ingredients in a skillet while continuously stirring.

5. Lay the salmon on top of a pile of broccoli or spinach.

6. Pour the sunflower butter sauce on top of the veggies and salmon.

7. Serve and enjoy while steaming hot.

Chicken Skin Crisps with Spicy Avocado Cream

Prep time: 5 min; **Cook time**: 20 min

Serving Size: 1 plate; **Serves**: 3

Calories: 66; **Total Fat**: 4 g; **Protein**: 7 g;

Total Carbs: 1 g; **Net Carbs**: 0 g; **Sugar**: 0 g; **Fiber**: 1 g;

Ingredients

- Skin from 3 to 4 pcs. of chicken thighs
- 1 ½ oz. of avocado pulp
- 1 ½ oz. of sour cream
- ½ pc. of jalapeño pepper, fresh, seeded & chopped finely
- ½ tsp. of sea salt

Instructions

1. Set oven to 350⁰ F and preheat.
2. Lay out the skins on a cookie sheet. Make sure they are as flat as possible.

3. Allow to bake for 12 to 15 minutes or until the skins become crispy and light brownish. Make sure they don't burn.

4. Take the skins from the cookie sheet and transfer to a paper towel. Allow to cool for a few minutes.

5. Combine the sour cream, avocado pulp, sea salt, and jalapeño in a small-sized bowl. Mix until everything is blended well.

6. Halve each piece of crispy chicken skin.

7. Put a Tbsp. of the avocado mix on top of each chicken skin.

8. Serve and enjoy immediately.

Sweet-Savory Baked Avocado w/ Coconut & Pecans

Prep time: 10 min; **Cook time**: 20 min

Serving Size: 1 plate; **Serves**: 2

Calories: 328; **Total Fat**: 33 g; **Protein**: 3 g;

Total Carbs: 10 g; **Net Carbs**: 2 g; **Sugar**: 1 g; **Fiber**: 8 g;

Ingredients

- 1 pc. of medium-sized avocado, skin on, halved & pitted

- 6 pcs. of pecan halves

- 2 Tbsp. of coconut oil

- 2. Tbsp. of unsweetened coconut, grated

Instructions

1. Set and pre-heat oven at 350⁰ F.

2. Place the avocado halves in a small-sized shallow baking dish, hole-side up.

3. Mix coconut oil with grated coconut in a small-sized bowl. Scoop the mixture into the avocado cavities.

4. Gently put 3 pecans at the top of the avocado halves.

5. Bake for about 20 minutes.

6. If cold dish is preferred, refrigerate first. Otherwise, serve and enjoy immediately.

Baked Avocado Crab Dynamite

Prep time: 10 min; **Cook time**: 20 min

Serving Size: 1 plate; **Serves**: 2

Calories: 217; **Total Fat**: 19 g; **Protein**: 7 g;

Total Carbs: 9 g; **Net Carbs**: 2 g; **Sugar**: 1 g; **Fiber**: 7 g;

Ingredients

- 1 medium-sized avocado, skin on, halved & pitted
- 1 ½ oz. of real crabmeat, no juices (drained)
- 1 tsp. of coconut aminos, tamari, or soy sauce
- 2 tsp. of mayonnaise
- ¼ tsp. of black pepper, freshly ground

Instructions

1. Pre-heat oven to 350⁰ F.

2. Place the avocado halves in a small-sized shallow baking dish, hole-side up.

3. Combine the crabmeat with mayonnaise, pepper, and coconut aminos in a small-sized bowl. Mix well.

4. Scoop the mixture into the avocado cavities.

5. Bake for about 20 minutes.

6. Dish is best served hot. Enjoy!

Spicy-Creamy Sesame Beef

Prep time: 10 min; **Cook time**: 30 min

Serving Size: 1 plate; **Serves**: 1

Calories: 518; **Total Fat**: 32 g; **Protein**: 53 g;

Total Carbs: 5 g; **Net Carbs**: 5 g; **Sugar**: 0 g; **Fiber**: 0 g;

Ingredients

- ½ lb. of 90% lean meat, ground
- Mexican spices or taco seasoning
- 2 oz. of hot pepper cheese, shredded
- 1 oz. of sour cream
- ½ Tbsp. of sesame seeds
- Water

Instructions

1. Cook the ground beef in a small-sized skillet until brown. Add a Tbsp. of water, or more, if necessary.

2. Sprinkle with a dash of taco seasoning or Mexican spices to taste.

3. Thoroughly mix. Allow to simmer for around 10 – 15 minutes.

4. Transfer the dish into a plate. Top the beef with shredded hot pepper cheese.

5. Combine the sour cream and sesame seeds for use as siding.

6. Immediately serve with sour cream mixture siding. If preferred, you can mix desired amount of the mixture with the dish to make the texture creamy.

THAI FISH W/ COCONUT & CURRY

Prep time: 10 min; **Cook time**: 20 min

Serving Size: 1; **Serves**: 5

Calories: 210; **Total Fat**: 33 g; **Protein**: 20 g;

Total Carbs: 5 g; **Net Carbs**: 5 g; **Sugar**: 0 g; **Fiber**: 0 g;

Ingredients

- 2 lbs. of white fish or salmon

- 5 Tbsp. of butter or ghee

- 1 can of coconut cream

- 2 Tbsp. of green or red curry paste

- 2/3 cup of cilantro, fresh & chopped

- Butter or olive oil to use for greasing the baking dish

Instructions

1. Set and pre-heat oven at 400⁰ F.

2. Grease a medium-sized, deep enough baking dish that can accommodate the fish. Put the fish in the dish.

3. Sprinkle some salt & pepper on the fish. Put a Tbsp. of butter on each pc. of fish.

4. Combine the curry paste, coconut cream, and cilantro in a small-sized bowl. Mix well and then spread over the fish.

5. Bake until well-done or around 20 minutes.

6. Serve and enjoy while hot. Best served with cooked rice or boiled veggies such as cauliflower and broccoli.

Chapter 5: Dessert Recipes

ALMOND BUTTER FUDGE

Prep time: 5 – 10 min; **Cook time**: 0

Serving Size: 1 cup; **Serves**: 12

Calories: 0; **Total Fat**: 12 g; **Protein**: 3 g;

Total Carbs: 3 g; **Net Carbs**: 3 g; **Sugar**: 0 g; **Fiber**: 0 g;

Ingredients

- 1 cup of unsweetened almond butter
- 1 cup of coconut oil
- ¼ cup of coconut milk
- 1 tsp. of vanilla extract
- Stevia (to sweeten/to taste)

Instructions

1. Combine the almond butter with coconut oil and melt until soft.

2. Put all the ingredients in a blender.

3. Process until everything is well-blended.

4. Pour the blended mixture into a baking pan.

5. Refrigerate for around 2 to 3 hours or until it sets.

6. Remove from the refrigerator and cut into around 12 pcs.

7. Serve and enjoy immediately.

Low Carb & Gluten-Free Bourbon Chocolate Truffles

Prep time: 15 min; **Cook time**: 0 min

Serving Size: 1 pc.; **Serves**: 12

Calories: 111; **Total Fat**: 10 g; **Protein**: 1.5 g;

Total Carbs: 4.5 g; **Net Carbs**: 1.5 g; **Sugar**: 0 g; **Fiber**: 3 g;

Ingredients

- 2 pcs. of avocado, ripe, skinned, & pitted
- ½ cup of premium cocoa powder
- 1 Tbsp. of heavy whipping cream
- 1 Tbsp. of granulated sugar substitute
- 2 Tbsp. of SF choco-flavored syrup
- 2 Tbsp. of bourbon (if desired)
- 2 Tbsp. coconut oil
- ½ cup of pecans, chopped

Instructions

1. Process all ingredients in in a food processor or blender, except the pecans, until a smooth consistency is achieved.

2. Chill the mixture until firm enough or around 1 hour.

3. Form 1″ balls from the mixture and roll each ball in the pecans. Refrigerate until the balls are firm.

4. Serve and enjoy!

Sugar-Free, Low Carb Chocolate Mousse

Prep time: 20 min; **Cook time**: 0 min

Serving Size: ½ cup; **Serves**: 8

Calories: 125; **Total Fat**: 12 g; **Protein**: 16 g;

Total Carbs: 2 g; **Net Carbs**: 2 g; **Sugar**: 0 g; **Fiber**: 0 g;

Ingredients

- 2 pcs avocados
- ½ cup of premium cocoa powder
- 2 Tbsp. of coconut oil
- 3 Tbsp. of sugar free chocolate flavored syrup
- 1 Tbsp. of heavy cream

Instructions

For the Pudding

1. Put all ingredients in the blender

2. Puree until consistency is smooth. Adjust the sweetness, as needed. If the mixture is too thick, add a bit of heavy

cream until the desired consistency for the pudding is achieved.

For the Mousse

1. Whip a cup of heavy cream with a tsp. of stevia sweetener until it becomes stiff.

2. If available, use a rubber spatula to fold 1/3 of the whipped cream gently into the pudding.

3. Fold the pudding mixture slowly into the remaining whipped cream until smooth and well-blended.

Notes: If you do not know what folding is, it is simply what it means literally. Just scoop from under the mixture and slowly "fold" or flip it together until blended. This is done to keep the fluffiness. If you just recklessly whip it, you will release air into the cream. Your work will wind up in a mess. Thus, it is important to fold gently.

ROSEMARY PANNA COTTA AND SOUR CREAM

Prep time: 30 min; **Cook time**: 7 min

Serving Size: 1 glass; **Serves**: 6

Calories: 332; **Total Fat**: 34 g; **Protein**: 3 g;

Total Carbs: 5 g; **Net Carbs**: 4 g; **Sugar**: 2 g; **Fiber**: 1 g;

Ingredients

- 1 ½ cups of sour cream
- 1 ½ cups of heavy whipping cream
- 2 medium-sized sprigs of rosemary, fresh & w/ extra leaves (for garnishing)
- 2 tsp. of unflavoured powdered gelatine
- 1 tsp. of sea salt

Instructions

1. Put the sour cream, heavy cream, and rosemary sprigs in a small-sized saucepan and cook at medium heat setting. Stir until everything melts and blends together.

2. Whisk the salt and gelatine in while continuously stirring

3. Reduce heat to low setting and allow to simmer for 4 minutes. Keep on stirring.

4. Take the rosemary sprigs out.

5. Pour the mixture into 6 small ramekins or glasses

6. Refrigerate for 6 hours or overnight until the mixture sets.

7. Remove from the refrigerator and garnish the glasses with rosemary leaves.

8. Serve and enjoy!

CREAMY LEMON BARS

Prep time: 30 min; **Cook time**: 0 min

Serving Size: 1 bar; **Serves**: 8

Calories: 333; **Total Fat**: 31 g; **Protein**: 13 g;

Total Carbs: 6 g; **Net Carbs**: 2 g; **Sugar**: 2 g; **Fiber**: 4 g;

Ingredients

- 4 oz. of melted butter

- 1 cup of pecans

- 3 oz. of unflavoured powdered gelatine

- 8 oz. of softened cream cheese

- ¼ cup of coconut flour

- 1 Tbsp. of lemon zest

- 2 Tbsp. of fresh lemon juice

- 1 cup of boiling water

- ¼ cup of granular Swerve

Instructions

1. Mix the pecans, melted butter, and coconut flour in a small-sized bowl.

2. Spread the mixture into an 8x8" baking dish or silicone glass. Set aside.

3. Put the gelatine in a medium-sized bowl with boiling water. Stir for around two minutes.

4. Add the rest of the ingredients into the bowl.

5. Thoroughly mix until all the lumps are gone.

6. Pour the mixture over the pecan crust.

7. Refrigerate to set.

8. Divide into 8 individual bars.

9. Best served chilled.

Dark Chocolate Orange Truffles

Prep time: 30 min; **Cook time**: 10 min (requires refrigeration after cooking)

Serving Size: 1 ball; **Serves**: 9

Calories: 78; **Total Fat**: 7 g; **Protein**: 1 g;

Total Carbs: 5 g; **Net Carbs**: 3 g; **Sugar**: 2 g; **Fiber**: 2 g;

Ingredients

For the Ganache

- 3 oz. of baking chocolate, unsweetened

- 2 Tbsp. of heavy cream

- 2 Tbsp. of confectioners Swerve

- ½ tsp. of liquid orange flavor

- 2 drops of stevia glycerite

- 1 Tbsp. of butter

For the Coating

- 2 tsp. of unsweetened cocoa powder

- 1 tsp. of confectioners Swerve

- 1 tsp. of orange zest, fresh

Instructions

1. Melt the chocolate over medium heat setting in a small-sized double boiler, while stirring slowly.

2. Add the butter, Swerve, cream, orange flavor, and stevia to the chocolate. Stir until everything is well-blended.

3. Take out of the heat. Continue to stir for around 10 seconds more.

4. Refrigerate the saucepan for around 1 hour or until the ganache congeals.

5. Use a spoon to scoop the ganache and make 9 balls from the mixture. Do this while wearing plastic gloves to keep the chocolate from sticking to your hands.

6. Create a coating powder by mixing the confectioners Swerve, orange zest and cocoa powder on a plate.

7. Thinly coat the ganache balls by rolling each ball through the coating powder.

8. To achieve the best consistency, refrigerate if the room temperature is over 70° F.

Gorgonzola Panna Cotta

Prep time: 20 min; **Cook time**: 5 min (requires refrigeration to set)

Serving Size: 1; **Serves**: 6

Calories: 435; **Total Fat**: 41 g; **Protein**: 14 g;

Total Carbs: 3 g; **Net Carbs**: 3 g; **Sugar**: 0 g; **Fiber**: 0 g;

Ingredients

- 12 oz. of crumbled Gorgonzola or blue cheese
- 12 pcs. of pecan halves
- 2 tsp. of powdered gelatine, unflavoured
- 1 ½ cups of heavy whipping cream

Instructions

1. Melt Gorgonzola and heavy cream in a small-sized saucepan for 2 minutes over medium heat setting. Remove the clots using a whisk.

2. Whisk the gelatine in until it is blended completely.

3. Pour the mixture into 6 small-sized ramekins or glasses evenly.

4. Refrigerate to set for 6 hours or overnight.

5. Garnish every glass w/ 2 pecan halves.

6. Serve and enjoy!

PUMPKIN PIE MOUSSE

Prep time: 15 min; **Cook time**: 0 min

Serving Size: 1; **Serves**: 3

Calories: 281; **Total Fat**: 28 g; **Protein**: 0 g;

Total Carbs: 6 g; **Net Carbs**: 5 g; **Sugar**: 3 g; **Fiber**: 1 g;

Ingredients

- 4 oz. cream cheese, softened
- 4 oz. of canned pumpkin purée
- ½ cup of heavy cream
- ½ tsp. of pumpkin pie spice
- ½ tsp. of cinnamon (for topping)
- 8 drops of liquid stevia
- ½ tsp. of vanilla extract

Instructions

1. Using a hand-held blender set on high, mix heavy cream in a small-sized mixing bowl until stiff peaks are formed.

2. Get a separate bowl and combine the pumpkin and cream cheese. Mix using a hand-held blender until consistency becomes smooth.

3. Fold the whipped cream until fully incorporated into the cheese mixture.

4. Put mousse in 3 separate serving dishes topped with cinnamon.

5. Serve and enjoy immediately. If desired, cover and refrigerate first before serving.

HERBS & GOAT CHEESE PANNA COTTA

Prep time: 20 min; **Cook time**: 10 min (requires refrigeration to set)

Serving Size: 1 glass; **Serves**: 6

Calories: 397; **Total Fat**: 38 g; **Protein**: 11 g;

Total Carbs: 3 g; **Net Carbs**: 3 g; **Sugar**: 2 g; **Fiber**: 0 g;

Ingredients

- ¾ cup of sour cream

- 1 ½ cups of heavy whipping cream

- 6 oz. goat cheese, soft

- 2 tsp. of unflavoured powdered gelatine

- 1 tsp. sea salt

- 1 tsp. of Herbes de Provence (available in most grocery stores)

Instructions

1. Combine the goat cheese, Herbes de Provence, heavy cream, and sour cream in a small-sized saucepan. Cook on medium heat setting. Stir constantly until the cheese melts.

2. Add salt and gelatine and whisk until everything is mixed completely.

3. Set heat to low and simmer for around 5 minutes while constantly stirring.

4. Pour the mixture into 6 small-sized glasses or ramekin evenly.

5. Refrigerate overnight or not less than 6 hours to set.

6. Serve in glasses. If preferred, dip glass in warm water first to loosen the panna cotta, and then invert the glass to transfer the contents to a small plate before serving.

7. Enjoy!

COCONUT BLUEBERRY CREAM BARS

Prep time: 20 min; **Cook time**: 5 min (requires refrigeration to set)

Serving Size: 1 bar; **Serves**: 20

Calories: 189; **Total Fat**: 20 g; **Protein**: 1 g;

Total Carbs: 3 g; **Net Carbs**: 3 g; **Sugar**: 3 g; **Fiber**: 0 g;

Ingredients

- 1 cup of fresh blueberries
- 8 oz. of butter
- ¾ cup of coconut oil
- 4 oz. of softened cream cheese, softened
- ¼ cup of coconut cream
- ¼ cup of granular Swerve

Instructions

1. Crush the blueberries gently in a small-sized bowl. Pour contents into an 8x8" glass or silicone baking dish.

2. Melt coconut oil and butter in a medium-sized saucepan over medium heat setting.

3. Take the dish away from heat. Allow to cook for around 5 minutes.

4. Put the remaining ingredients in the saucepan. Mix thoroughly using a wooden spoon.

5. Top the blueberries with the mixture. Put them in the freezer to set.

6. Take the saucepan out of the freezer and let it warm up a bit for around 15 minutes.

7. Cut the dish into 20 bars of equal size.

8. Serve and enjoy!

Panna Cotta Infused w/ Turmeric

Prep time: 20 min; **Cook time**: 8 min (requires refrigeration to set)

Serving Size: 1 glass; **Serves**: 6

Calories: 130; **Total Fat**: 12 g; **Protein**: 4 g;

Total Carbs: 3 g; **Net Carbs**: 3 g; **Sugar**: 0 g; **Fiber**: 0 g;

Ingredients

- 1 ½ cups of beef stock, homemade
- 1 ½ cups of coconut milk, refrigerated and water separated from cream
- 1 Tbsp. of turmeric
- ½ tbsp. of sea salt
- 1 ½ Tbsp. of unflavored powdered gelatin

Instructions

1. Heat the beef stock and coconut cream in a small-sized saucepan over medium heat setting.

2. Gradually whisk the gelatine in until it is completely incorporated.

3. Add some salt and turmeric, then allow to simmer for about 5 minutes.

4. Divide the mixture equally among 6 small-sized glasses or ramekins.

5. Refrigerate to set for 6 hours or overnight.

6. The dessert is best served and enjoyed cold.

Low-Fat Peach Cobblers (Sugar-Free)

Prep time: 5 min; **Cook time**: 15 min

Serving Size: 1 cup; **Serves**: 4

Calories: 80; **Total Fat**: 0.4 g; **Protein**: 6 g;

Total Carbs: 13.5 g; **Net Carbs**: 13 g; **Sugar**: 0 g; **Fiber**: 0.5 g;

Ingredients

- ¼ cup of Heart Smart Bisquick

- 1 large-sized egg

- ½ cup of skim milk

- 1 tsp. of Splenda

- 8 oz. of Del Monte Lite Peaches (diced and drained)

Instructions

1. Drain diced peaches and separate into 4 oven-safe, individual dessert cups.

2. Place Bisquick, egg, Splenda, and skim milk in a small-sized bowl, then mix well.

3. Pour ¼ of the mixture on top of each peach cup.

4. Bake for around 15 minutes at 400 degrees or until the topping turns brown.

5. Can be served hot or cold.

Cheesy Prosciutto Cup Muffin

Prep time: 20 min; **Cook time**: 12 min

Serving Size: 1 muffin; **Serves**: 1

Calories: 218; **Total Fat**: 15 g; **Protein**: 18 g;

Total Carbs: 2 g; **Net Carbs**: 2 g; **Sugar**: 0 g; **Fiber**: 0 g;

Ingredients

- 1 slice (1/2 oz.) of prosciutto

- 1 medium-sized egg yolk

- ½ oz. grated Parmesan cheese

- ½ oz. Brie cheese, diced

- 1/3 oz. mozzarella cheese, diced

Instructions

1. Set and pre-heat oven at 400⁰ F.

2. Get a muffin tin that has around 1 ½″ deep and 2 ½″ wide hole.

3. Fold the prosciutto in half to make it squarish.

4. Put it in the muffin tin hole to completely line it.

5. Put the egg yolk in the prosciutto cup.

6. Gently top the egg yolk with the cheeses to avoid breaking the yolk.

7. Bake for approximately 12 minutes or until the yolk is warmed and cooked, but still runny.

8. Allow the muffin to cool for around 10 minutes before taking out of the muffin pan.

9. Serve and enjoy!

CHOCOLATE CHIA PUDDING

Prep time: 20 min; **Cook time**: 0 min

Serving Size: 1 cup; **Serves**: 4

Calories: 277; **Total Fat**: 27 g; **Protein**: 3 g;

Total Carbs: 14 g; **Net Carbs**: 12 g; **Sugar**: 2 g; **Fiber**: 2 g;

Ingredients

- ¼ cup of chia seeds
- 1 cup of heavy cream
- 2 Tbsp. of granular Swerve or erythritol
- 2 Tbsp. of cocoa powder
- 1 Tbsp. of chocolate chips, sugar-free

Instructions

1. Set aside the chocolate chips, then mix the rest of the ingredients in a medium-sized bowl. Allow the mixture to sit for no less than 15 minutes, while stirring occasionally.

2. Divide equally among 4 cups.

3. Garnish each cup with the chocolate chips previously set aside.

4. Dessert is best enjoyed cold. It may be refrigerated for a maximum of 3 days.

Salty PB Cup Fudge

Prep time: 5 min; **Cook time**: 8 min

Serving Size: 1; **Serves**: 12

Calories: 150; **Total Fat**: 15 g; **Protein**: 3 g;

Total Carbs: 3 g; **Net Carbs**: 2 g; **Sugar**: 1 g; **Fiber**: 1 g;

Ingredients

- ½ cup of coconut oil
- ½ cup of almond butter
- 3 Tbsp. of cocoa powder
- 1 Tbsp. of vanilla extract
- 12 drops of liquid stevia
- 1 tsp. of coarse sea salt

Instructions

1. Heat a small-sized saucepan over medium setting. Melt the coconut oil and almond butter together.

2. Add the vanilla, cocoa powder, and stevia. Blend well by stirring.

3. Get a silicone candy mold and fill 12 slots with the mixture. Alternatively, you can use an ice cube tray with a silicone bottom.

4. Refrigerate to set for 2 hours or more.

5. Serve cold.

Conclusion

Thank you once more for buying and reading this book.

I hope you have gained a better understanding and appreciation for the ketogenic diet and what it can do for your overall health and well-being.

Hopefully, by trying out some of the recipes in this book, you will be inspired to create your own. The next step is to practice what you have learned from the book and incorporate some of the ketogenic diet recipes featured here on a daily basis to enjoy all the health benefits from the diet.

Finally, if you enjoyed this book, then I'd like to ask you for a favor, would you be kind enough to leave a review for this book on Amazon? It'd be greatly appreciated!

Please leave a review at: www.amazon.com/dp/B06XYG9CVT

Thanks again for getting a copy of this book. Good luck!